How to Start the Paleo Diet Today:

Eating Primal the Way You're Supposed To

Introduction

I want to thank you and congratulate you for downloading the book, *"How to start the Paleo diet today: Eating Primal the Way you're supposed to."*

This book contains proven steps and strategies on how to start living the Paleo diet. The first chapter gives you a detailed explanation of what the Paleo diet is. The following two chapters will provide you with detailed information of food that you should eat and food that you should not eat. The next chapter gives you a systematic and practical guide into changing your current diet to the Paleo diet. The final chapter highlights the challenges that you may encounter during the transition to the Paleo diet and how to overcome them.

By the time you finish reading the last sentence, you will have the confidence needed to start the Paleo diet immediately!

Thanks again for downloading this book, I hope you enjoy it!

Chapter 1: What is the Paleo diet?

The Paleo diet, also called the Caveman diet, the Stone Age diet, or the Primal diet, is a diet that involves eating what our ancestors of the Paleolithic era ate. During this time, some plants and animals were yet to be domesticated. In addition, there were no factories and the knowhow available to produce processed food. Our ancestors were yet to discover sugar, salt and other commonly used spices. Although you might think that the Paleo diet is a new thing, it has been in existence since 40 years ago!

Why would anyone adopt the Paleo diet?

You might consider going Paleo if you want to lose weight, acquire more muscle, reduce body fat, and escape from the modern conditions associated with dietary habits. Such conditions include high blood pressure, arthritis, diabetes, and autoimmune diseases. Nonetheless, you have to do it the right way: there are controversies about what food is ancient and used by the cave dweller and what quantities of this food are healthy and beneficial to your body. The Paleo diet at times contradicts with other conventional food diets such as being a vegetarian diet.

Although the Paleo diet might help you lose weight, always remember that it is not one of the fad diets. All the same, you need to approach this option with care in order to be healthy and reap maximum benefits from the diet. Always consult with your doctor before starting a diet of any kind. The following chapters highlight the most important aspects of the Paleo diet and will demystify modern myths about the Paleo diet to help you make a smooth transition from your routine diet to Paleo diet.

In the contemporary world, there are different versions of the Paleo diet. As a beginner, you might be confused about which of these versions is the best. This book will give you guidance in adopting a Paleo diet that is realistic, simple, and convenient for you.

Chapter 2: Components of the Paleo Diet

The Paleo diet primarily involves eating that which the Caveman ate in the Paleolithic era. The diet consists of foods that are high in protein and low in carbohydrates.

Proteins

You should eat a lot of protein: more than the one recommended by health experts. Health experts recommend that you take 10-35% of calories derived from proteins. In contrast, if you are going the Paleo way, you have to take about 19-35 % of calories derived from proteins.

Carbohydrates

You should take a few carbohydrates derived from fresh fruits and vegetables that lack starch. These should make up approximately 35-45% calories of carbohydrates every day. Health experts recommend that the carbohydrates you take comprise 45 to 65 %

of the total calorie intake. In the contemporary diet, grains and dairy products contribute the largest proportion of carbohydrates. To adapt to the Paleo diet, you will have to do away with grains and dairy products as these were not available in the Paleolithic era and did not qualify to be part of the Paleo diet.

Fiber

The Paleo diet includes high fiber content derived from vegetables and fruits that lack starch. Despite the high content of fiber in grains, do not take them, as they are not part of the Paleo diet.

Fat

You should take many polyunsaturated and monosaturated fats such as omega-3 fats in larger proportions than before. However, you should avoid trans-fats such as omega-6 fats.

Salt

As aforementioned, our ancestors of the Paleolithic era were yet to discover salt. For this reason, salt is not included in the Paleo diet.

Vitamins and Minerals

The diet does includes large intake of vitamins derived from animals that primarily feed on grass and vegetables but not grains.

The Paleo diet is high in protein, fiber, fat, vitamins and minerals, but low in carbohydrates and salt.

Chapter 3: Food you should eat

In order to obtain the above components in the required proportions, you have to select your food wisely. The following are foods that you should regularly take.

1. Seafood, Eggs and Meat

Flesh (animal and fish) will provide you with the highest calorie content of the Paleo diet. You should ensure that you select high-quality sources of proteins for this category of food. Although wild meat and salmon may be a bit expensive, cheaper options such as fresh or frozen salmon, organic chicken and grass-fed beef are available.

Make sure the livestock meat you purchase is grass-fed, organic and does not contain antibiotics. Livestock meat includes lamb, pork and beef. You should also consume game meat such as boar meat and deer meat. When purchasing meat, always ensure that you get lean cuts rather than meat with high fat content.

The poultry you take should be organic and free of hormones. Options include Cornish hens, goose, turkey, chicken and duck. Ensure that the eggs you include in your diet come from organic and free-range birds.

You should consume a variety of seafood such as oysters, lobsters, clams, crab, shrimp, fish and other mollusks and crustaceans. You should focus on cold-water fish like salmon, haddock, mackerel and cod to obtain maximum omega-3 fats.

How do you prepare your seafood or animal flesh?

You can steam, boil, grill, bake, broil or pan-fry your seafood or meat. Do not deep-fry your food since butter and deep frying oils are not included in the Paleo diet.

2.Plant-based fats

You should take fats derived from plants. Avocados, olive oil and olives are the options. Prepare food from fats derived from these plants in place of butter —a dairy product. You should use pure olive oil in cooking and extra virgin olive oil or grape-seed for dressing salads.

3.Seeds and nuts

Take all nuts except peanuts. Nuts made a big proportion of the diet of the hunter-gatherers humans of the Paleolithic era. Although peanuts have the suffix "nuts," they are only nuts by name. They fall under the same category of food as beans and peas and you should not consume such. You should take seeds such as sunflower seeds, sesame seeds, flax seeds, pumpkin seeds and other seeds. Do not worry about having to get rid of pasta and rice from your diet; quinoa makes a great substitute for barley, rice, pasta and other common grains.

4.Fruits and Vegetables

You should concentrate on consuming fruits that were not cultivated before adoption of agricultural techniques. Such fruits include berries such as strawberries, blueberries, cranberries and raspberries. You should also take fruits that grow on trees such as apples, pears, nectarines, cherries, plums, citrus fruits and peaches.

Vegetables that you should take include carrots and onions. However, take carrots moderately because they have a high glycemic index.

Always aim at consuming low-glycemic vegetables and fruits to get a steady supply of energy and maintain an even blood sugar level.

You should go for the best quality when shopping for fruits and vegetables. Look for vegetables and fruits that have been grown organically. Also purchase that which is in season; you will be assured of freshness and low cost. If you take frozen fruits and vegetables, do not do so regularly. Do not take canned fruits and vegetables because they have high contents of salt.

5.Condiments

Some condiments are part of the Paleo diet while others are not. Only condiments that have no added sugar or some forbidden ingredients are part of the Paleo diet. Do not take ketchup. You should focus your attention on herbs and spices instead of condiments. However, you should consume the mustard—a product from seeds that contains no added sugar.

6.Drinks

You should consume vegetable and fruit juices but in moderation to maintain a constant blood sugar level. You could take tea and coffee but do not use dairy milk or sugar in them. Instead, use almond milk and honey to improve to bring them to your preferred taste.

Chapter 4: Food that you should not eat

If you are looking forward to reaping maximum benefits from the Paleo diet, you should avoid foods that stimulate storage of fats, increase blood sugar and hinder metabolism. You should not take the following types of food.

Grains

Grains such as barley, oats, pasta, rice and bread are not part of the Paleo diet simply because they are cultivated produce. Grains are carbohydrates in nature so when they are digested they become glucose which is the primary source of energy in the body. If your body fails to use all of the glucose released from the digestion of grains, it converts it to fat for storage. It is, therefore, the main cause of obese and overweight in majority of people. In addition, grains have dire consequences. Grains contain lectins and gluten. Gluten is a protein packed in grains such as barley, wheat and rye. Most individuals are gluten-intolerant and are prone to conditions such as reproductive problems, acid reflux, joint pain and dermatitis.

Lectin, on the other hand, is a natural toxin present in most grains. Scientifically, lectin is an evolution of grains to prevent them from consumption by humans and other animals and hence ensure their continued survival and completion of their life cycles. Lectin is harmful to the well-being of human beings because it impairs the normal repair of the gastrointestinal tract from wear and tear. The damaged tract fails to absorb digested food properly and a myriad of medical conditions may ensue.

Dairy

Did your Paleolithic ancestors keep cows? Of course, they did not. Dairy in Paleo diet is a controversial issue. The majority of people are lactose intolerant.

It could imply that the human body has not yet evolved to recognize milk as food.

Casein intolerance is another issue that points to the fact that the human body is yet to recognize milk as food. Did you know that casein is structurally similar to gluten? Yes, it is. It, like gluten, has adverse effects on the alimentary canal. Casein causes the shredding of the intestinal wall causing the immune system to launch an attack on the wall. It therefore causes autoimmune diseases that can lead to death.

Overall, you already know that of all animals, only human beings continue to take milk after their infancy. Your paleo ancestors did not keep cows and only babies consumed milk. For this reason, milk and milk products do not qualify to be part of the Paleo diet.

Stem Tubers

You probably have heard that the potato is a Paleo food. Nonetheless, you should not eat potato and other stem tubers in large proportions. Such food types cause blood sugar to skyrocket to very high levels shortly after consumption which will then drastically fall back down after a short while. This drastic fall of blood sugar below the initial level is not healthy and leaves you feeling awful. Potato derived food and other stem tubers have high glycemic indices that are close to that of refined sugar. If you eat potatoes, your blood sugar will shoot up and, consequently, your blood insulin concentration will go up as well. If this frequently occurs then you will become insulin resistant.

Insulin resistance predisposes you to a number of conditions collectively known as the metabolic syndrome. They include cardiovascular disease, high blood cholesterol, obesity, type 2 diabetes, hypertension and other abnormalities such as skin tags, breast cancer, colon cancer, prostate cancer, systemic inflammation, gout and acne.

Highly processed food

Do not consume French fries, ice cream, hamburgers, pizzas and other fast foods, frozen meals and sweet, salty snacks. These types of food contain high sugar and salt content and do not qualify to be in the Paleo diet.

Alcohol

Do not take alcohol at all. Alcohol was not in existence in the Paleolithic era. In addition, it has a lot of sugar, has low calories and low nutritional value to benefit the body. Alcohol also has the dire effects of dehydrating your body.

Legumes

Legumes also contain lectin and thus require one to cook them for long hours or soak them for fermentation. The most toxic is kidney and soybeans when eaten uncooked. A few uncooked kidney beans trigger symptoms of food poisoning. Beans that are undercooked have high toxicity too. Raw peanuts contain molds and fungus. Regardless of the toxicity of beans, the fact is that they were not food for the Paleolithic generation and should not be part of the Paleo diet in the first place.

Sugar

Do not make sugar a part of your diet. If you avoid sugar then you will achieve low blood sugar and reduce your chances of becoming diabetic. Do not substitute sugar with artificial sweeteners too as they are high in calories. Instead, use honey to sweeten your beverages.

Chapter 5: Do it today! Start the Paleo diet

Now that you know what you can and cannot eat, it is time you start your new life the Caveman way. You should follow the following practical steps for an easy transition.

1. Do a kitchen makeover

Now that you know what you should eat and what you should not eat, take time to get rid of that, which is not Paleo. Get rid of all processed food and empty your trashcan immediately.

2. Go out and shop for groceries

Now that your kitchen is almost empty, fill it with the healthy, natural foods that you are going to eat from now on. You can rely on the food list of Paleo food. Remember to pick the fresh vegetables, fruits, grass-fed beef, salmon and other healthy Paleo foods.

While you are shopping spend more time on the grocery section, you should avoid ingredients. Avoid temptation to buy seasonings. However, you can take one type of seasoning as you gradually progress to a life without seasoned food.

3.Learn to cook

You should have known by now that not many eateries or restaurants offer the Paleo diet. You will have no option but to make most of your meals at home. You must learn to cook the natural foods and maintain quality. Learn to cook to bring out the natural flavor of different foods; remember that seasoning in Paleo diet is rare. You can purchase cookbooks of the Paleo diet and recipes. Who knows? You might even discover that you have an innate talent in cooking!

Start the road to your new life with easy to make recipes and continue to progress to complex ones.

The more recipes you have, the more choices of meals you will have at your disposal.

4.Exercise

You will reap maximum benefits from the Paleo diet if you have an active life. Are you trying to lose those extra pounds and become fit? Are you trying to avoid lifestyle diseases? Be aware that the Paleo diet is not enough. The Cavemen were very active and barely had time to rest. They would walk in search of fruits, chase animals in search of meat and run away from predators. You need to be physically active even if that means taking a walk, jogging, swimming and gardening. You could effortlessly achieve this by simply walking to your place of work.

5.Sleep

Sleep is essential for good health. You will need a good sleep to allow your body to relax after an active day. You will gain the following from sleep:

- Increased energy

- Improved moods

- Effective immune system

- Relief from stress

- Increased memory

- Decreased chances of developing diabetes, obesity and heart disease

- If you are an athlete, you will notice an improvement in your performance

How do you get a better sleep?

You get a good sleep by properly preparing yourself for sleep. Draw the curtains, switch off all the electronics and try to sleep at the same time and wake up at the same time on a daily basis.

Chapter 6: Challenges as a Paleo diet beginner

Once you begin the transition to the Paleo diet, you will realize that it is not a walk in the park. You will have to face and overcome several challenges presented by your body's response to the change as well as those around you.

Your body will go through a cleansing period in the first two weeks. It will also change from using sugar as the main energy source and start using fat instead. You may experience undesirable side effects such as sugar craving, mood swings and fatigue.

You will have problems with your friends and family; remember that you have probably made the transition alone. You will be tempted to go back to your former lifestyle if you do not stand your ground.

How do you treat friends and family during the transition?

a)Always remain positive.

Do not rush to say what you cannot eat. Instead, mention that which you can eat. If you are quick to say what you cannot eat, you will raise an argument with those around you who choose to eat that type of food. You should keep calm and let everyone chose whatever they like.

b)Do not go keep bragging

You do not have to go telling everyone your new diet. With time, they will be asking you to disclose the secret! It will save you from ridicule and discouragement at the beginning of your transition.

c)Research

Do not relax and assume you know it all. You should research on the internet and get as much information as you can about the Paleo diet. It is only through the research that you will know what different foods contribute to the well being of your body. It is also through researching that you will learn what to expect with that kind of food, the different challenges and possible solutions to these challenges.

How do you to cope with your body's reaction during transition?

You might suffer from digestive distress—a condition caused by low Hydrochloric (HCL) acid in the stomach, reduced release of digestive enzymes and inflammation of the gut. Low HCL could be due to the presence of *Helicobacter pylori*. You should go for the test to confirm if you have the bacteria or not. You can simply correct low stomach acid by taking HCL alongside proteases such as pepsin. It solves not only the problem of low stomach acid, but also the problem of reduced enzyme production since HCL triggers production of digestive enzymes.

Alternatively, you could take bitter herbs to stimulate HCL production in your stomach. Studies have shown that bitter herbs increase the flow of juices involved in digestion such as HCL, pancreatic enzymes, pepsin, bile and gastric juice. You should try the following herbs predominantly used in China and the Western regions.

- Ginger
- beet root
- goldenseal root
- milk thistle
- yellow dock
- peppermint Fennel
- Dandelion and
- gentian root

If you have an inflamed gut, you should stop consumption of foods with insoluble fiber. You should reduce the proportion and variety of vegetables you take until you notice some improvement.

You might experience fatigue, lightheadedness, agitation and even loss of concentration. You might have strong craving for sugar too. These are issues relating to what you are eating. Your body will slowly adjust to the new lifestyle. However, there are things you can do to ease the transition. Take food rich in riboflavin and carnitine. The two substances ease in energy production from fats and hence reduce fatigue and sluggishness. Take food rich in magnesium, chromium and biotin; these three macronutrients aid in sugar balance and hence prevent you from developing sugar cravings. Cope with sugar imbalance by eating high protein food more often if you have low blood sugar and eating low-carbohydrate content frequently if you have high blood sugar.

Conclusion

Thank you again for downloading this book!

I hope this book was able to help you start the Paleo diet and a healthier, happier life!

The next step is to maintain this new diet and life. Don't be afraid to explore other Paleo foods not described here in this book.

Finally, if you enjoyed this book, would you be kind enough to leave a review for this book on Amazon? It'd be greatly appreciated!

www.ingramcontent.com/pod-product-compliance
Lightning Source LLC
Chambersburg PA
CBHW062031280526
45787CB00005B/2285